Ketogenic Diet

A Quick Low Carb Guide For Busy People To Rapid Weight Loss & Healthy Eating Mastery

What This Book Has For You

I want to thank you and congratulate you for buying the book *"Ketogenic Diet: A Quick Low Carb Guide For Busy People To Rapid Weight Loss & Healthy Eating Mastery"*.

This guide is about the popular "Ketogenic Diet", which is a proven method of successful weight loss and overall health improvement. The diet has a unique structure which makes it a high-fat, low-carb nutritional method. According to some of the best nutritionists and chefs around the world, Ketogenic diet is not only a diet but a way of life.

The diet is considered an effective regimen that is also associated with a number of health benefits. It is not only producing healthy weight loss results, but can help with a number of other health conditions discussed in detail. The diet focuses on adding more real food to your life and staying in ketosis.

This kind of diet is known for shifting your body habits from being a sugar-burner to becoming a fat-burner – thus improving and supporting better health and lifestyle. It has also shown great results in improving health issues from obesity to epilepsy to autoimmune diseases and more.

It is very important to have the right mindset and approach for Ketogenic diet. Most people delay getting on this healthier lifestyle journey, just because they think they are too lazy or have an extremely packed schedule to work this diet out. If that sounds like you, don't stress about learning how to adjust your body with your diet, because you are just about to read this amazing book.

This book does not only include simple and delicious recipes, but information about Ketogenic diet that will help you keep up with it and benefit from it. It will make it easier for you to prepare delicious, nutrient-rich, and quick Ketogenic meals that you can enjoy guilt-free.

This book will also help you understand how you can gain energy and lose weight without relying on sugar and other high-carb food. It will make following this diet easy and accessible for everyone, regardless of how caught up you are with your schedule...plus it is a great start for beginners who are just beginning to learn about this amazing Ketogenic diet!

Thanks again for buying this book, I hope you enjoy it!

Table of Contents

Chapter 1: What Is Ketogenic Diet And How Can It Help You Lose Weight?

It is extremely important for everyone to have a good know-how about this powerful tool – Ketogenic Diet – in order to lose weight and achieve optimal health before beginning. The Ketogenic Diet offers a number of health benefits including sustainable weight loss, because of its unique formulation that helps the body shift its approach. This diet is a high-fat, low-carb that brings a big metabolic change to improve overall wellbeing.

More than 20 studies prove that the diet has amazing and long lasting results in weight loss and overall health improvement. Ketogenic is a diet that more nutritionists suggest, as it does not only help with weight loss, but also offers great benefits against cancer, diabetes, Alzheimer's disease and epilepsy.

If you are a beginner and don't know how to go about implementing this positive change in your life, go through and learn about everything ketogenic diet contains.

This diet is also termed as "Keto". It focuses on increasing high-fat content together with reducing the carb intake. For this reason, it is is also sometimes confused with low-carb and Atkins diets.

Ketogenic diet involves reducing the consumption of carbohydrates drastically and replacing that with fat. The sudden change in your eating pattern will put your body into a metabolic state known as ketosis.

With this change, the body also shifts its behavior towards burning sugar for energy. In fact, it starts using the fat content for producing energy. The fat is then turned into ketones in the liver, which is responsible for supping energy to the brain.

There are also a number of health and hormonal benefits of adopting this lifestyle. When ketone levels increase in the body, it also leads to reduction in insulin and blood sugar levels. This in itself contains a number of health benefits, which will be covered in this book.

For easy understanding, for now just remember that ketogenic diet is all about high-fat and low-carb consumption. It reduces the insulin level of the body and alters the metabolism structure of the body away from carbs and towards ketones and fats.

Ketogenic Diet and Weight Loss

Ketogenic diet is a proven method for successful weight loss. The best part about this diet is that it does not only fight obesity – which is becoming one of the major reasons for a number of health issues – but is also associated with a number of other diseases.

Research has shown that ketogenic diet is way superior to the average low-fat diets that people often follow. It is easier to follow, because it is extremely filling. The satiation level is higher and there's less craving for foods that are not allowed. Even though the diet fills you up, it still manages to help you lose weight without really tracking your food or paying attention to the calories.

Another study showed how volunteers who followed the ketogenic diet helped them lose 2.2 times more than other people following the regular low-fat, calorie-restricted diet. The results also showed improvement in the HDL cholesterol and triglyceride in the body.

There are several other reasons why this diet is superior to other regular low-fat and low-calorie diets. The protein intake also increases naturally, which further leads to great benefits.

Other Amazing Health Benefits Of Ketogenic Diet

There is a long list of health benefits associated with ketogenic diet. It is highly recommended that you get a blood lipid panel done before you begin following the plan. This will help you compare results after a month of switching to this diet.

- **Freedom from sugar cravings, food fixations and hypoglycemic_** – It is one of the best benefits you can experience. Having a control over your eating pattern is highly empowering, which can offer you great weight loss benefits.

- **Controlled blood pressure** – Diets that are low in carbs are naturally very effective at keeping a control over your blood pressure. If you have been on medications for lowering blood pressure, be aware that the same medication could make you feel dizzy if you continue taking them after switching your diet to ketogenic plan. Speak to your doctor and get your medicine adjusted.

- **Lack of hunger** – The diet enhances ketone bodies, which dampen the appetite. The fat fills you up and keeps you satisfied. You will have less hunger pangs and forgetting to eat may become a norm. You will be amazed with this change, especially if you have been struggling with your food cravings and addiction issues.

- **Drop in cholesterol** – A diet rich in excess glucose leads to cholesterol problems. Once your sugar intake drops down, inflammation level drops too causing less damage to your arterial system. As a result, the cholesterol level reduces too since your body has less glucose to make it.

- **More Energy** – If you have been experiencing chronic fatigue symptoms, switching to a ketogenic diet will improve the condition. You will be surprised at your energy levels.

- **Weight loss** – Following a ketogenic diet plan also offers great weight loss benefits. However, if your fasting insulin level is high, you might want to add strenuous workout to your routine. High intensity training improves the insulin sensitivity level of your muscles and decreases the level of fasting insulin. This leads to further weight loss.

Other benefits include improved digestion, relief from heartburn and gum disease, and better mood stabilization. But the key to experiencing the list of these benefits is to take a proper ketogenic diet that is based on low carbs, high natural fats and moderate protein.

The problem occurs when the fat is combined with a lot of carbohydrates. The sugar level from carbohydrates can get you into trouble. This combination will not benefit you with weight loss, instead will lead to weight gain. As a result, you may even experience other health problems that are associated with high carb diet.

Therefore, it is very important to understand this breakdown to avoid problems. Keep reading!

Your Guide to Protein, Carb and Fats

A healthy ketogenic diet is based on three key factors:

1. **Determine your ideal body weight.** You can use online body weight calculators to determine your ideal weight according to your gender, height and age. In case you don't want to get into those details, select a body weight where you feel best.

2. **Establish a calorie requirement on a daily basis to maintain that body weight.** The best way to calculate the calorie requirement is by using this handy calculator https://www.bcm.edu/cnrc-apps/caloriesneed.cfm. Your current weight, ideal weight and activity level will help you figure out the daily calorie amount that should be consumed to maintain that weight or normal Body Mass Index (BMI).

3. **Figure out the amount of carb, protein and fat to eat following the ketogenic diet.** The guidelines below, your daily caloric intake and ideal body weight will help you figure out your intake of carbohydrates, protein, and fat in calorie and gram measure.

The Gram Guide

Here's your gram guide to make your ketogenic diet a success!

Protein Requirement

Following a ketogenic diet, your protein intake should be between 1g and 1.5g for every kilogram of your ideal body weight or lean body mass.

For example, if your weight is 150lb and has a lean body mass of 100lb, then the optimal intake of protein should be between 45g to 67.5g.

Here's the math:

100lb of lean body mass = 45kg

45kg x 1g = 45g of protein

45kg x 1.5g = 67.5g of protein

It is important to keep up with that range. Every gram of protein has 4 calories, which means that 45-67.5g will be 180-272 calories. That should be your daily intake.

Carbohydrate Requirement

The goal of ketogenic diet is to keep your daily carbohydrate count under 60 grams. However, this is also a subjective thing. If your body has increased levels of muscle mass and exercise a lot, you can probably afford to eat more carbs and stay in ketosis.

On the other hand, if you are diabetic, have insulin resistant and have other metabolic issues, you might have to further cut down on carbohydrates. In case your only goal is to lose weight following the ketogenic diet, your carbohydrate intake should go even lower than 30g per day. In case you are not able to lose weight after cutting down on your carbohydrates, you may need to bring down your protein towards the 1g/kg range, but don't go less than that.

If that does not work either, you might need to reduce your fat intake until you start losing weight again.

Fat Requirements

This is the most important part of the plan. Calories from oils and natural fats will keep up with balancing your calories after subtracting carb and protein calories. This is the most important part to determine before you start with this plan.

Keep reading to learn how fat grams should be determined to make ketogenic diet work for you like magic.

Chapter 2: Putting Everything Together

To make sure the ketogenic diet works, it is important to put all the steps together. The following example will help you understand how to make the most out of ketogenic diet to gain maximum benefits.

For example: an overweight individual is aiming to get down to an ideal weight of 150 pounds. The calorie limit for that person is 1800 in a day – 30g of carbs and 1g/kg.

First and foremost, get the weight in kilograms. Simply divide your weight in pounds by 2.2 to do the math. Both carbs and protein have 4 calories in one gram and fat has 9 calories in one gram. Therefore, to achieve 1800 calories, you will need to adjust it like this:

Protein: convert 150 pounds into kilograms. Protein intake should be 150/2.2 = 68kg. For the lowest count 68x1g = 68g or 272 calories

Carbohydrates: 30 grams = 120 calories

Total number of calories from protein and carbohydrates = 392 calories.

Fat grams will be determined from balance of total calories = 1800 total calories (minus) total number of calories (from protein and carb).

1800 – 329 = 1408 fat calories.

This shows that 1408 calories from the daily calorie count should be based on fat. To get the amount in grams, divide 1408 calories by 9 (calorie in each gram of fat) = 156g.

This concludes that 156g of fat can be consumed by the individual to achieve the daily 1800 calories for weight loss.

Now calculate your protein, carb, and fat intake according to the number of calories you can eat on daily basis.

General Guidelines and Rules – Planning Out Your Shopping List

The following are some rules and guidelines for following a ketogenic diet to deliver you successful results. The best way to get more benefits from this diet is to stick to whatever is mentioned below. All other aspects of this diet are flexible.

Rule 1 –Add only the foods mentioned in this book to your diet.

In case you want to add other foods, check the label carbohydrate content and carefully check for the serving size too. Whatever you decide to consume should have 2 grams or less per serving for dairy or meat products, or 5 grams or less for vegetables.

Rule 2 –When it is time to eat, make your choice from the food items listed follows. This list should also make your shopping list.

Stop eating once the hunger subsides.

Meats, seafood, poultry (frozen or fresh, check for additives before using):

✓ Different kinds of meat –lamb, beef, goat, veal, wild game. It is preferable to eat grass fed meat only since the fatty acid profile of such meat is better.

✓ Pork –Boston butt, pork loin, ham, pork chops. Watch for added sugar.

✓ Canned salmon or tuna are acceptable, but don't forget to check out the labels for added fillers and sugars.

✓ Fish or any kind of seafood, preferably wild caught: calamari, bass, anchovies, cod, catfish, halibut, flounder, mackerel, herring, mahi-mahi, sardines, salmon, scrod, scallops, snapper, sole, tuna, and trout.

✓ Poultry: chicken, quail, turkey, duck, Cornish hen, pheasant, goose.

✓ Shellfish: crab, clams, lobster, shrimp, scallops, mussels, squid, oysters.

✓ Sausage and bacon: check labels to determine carb level. Less than 2g per serving allowed.

✓ Whole eggs: eggs can be prepared using different methods: fried, deviled, hard-boiled, scrambled, poached, omelet, soft-boiled.

✓ Soy products including tempeh, edamame, and tofu are some good options and excellent as protein sources.

However, they are also high in carbs so better use them carefully.

✓ Avoid foods which include whey protein until you have achieved your weight loss goal. The ingredient is said to spike insulin.

All the protein sources mentioned above can be cooked in a microwave, baked, grilled, sautéed, stir-fried, fried, and roasted using natural fats. Using cornmeal, breading or flour for coating is not allowed.

Rule 3 –It is important to eat salad greens every day. Add one or two cups of salad greens and one cup of fibrous vegetables to your daily meal. This will ensure your vitamin K intake is appropriate.

Salad greens can be consumed 1-2 cups every day. 1 cup equals a fist-size potion. Choose your salad greens from the following:

✓ Chives

✓ Cabbage (all varieties)

✓ Lettuce (all varieties)

✓ Spinach

✓ Parsley

✓ Kale

✓ Parsley

✓ Chard

✓ Greens (all varieties including collards, beet, turnip, and mustard)

Consume 1 cup of fibrous vegetables in a day. You can pick from the following a single choice or combine a few to make your portion.

✓ Asparagus

✓ Alfalfa and bean sprouts

✓ Okra

✓ Radishes

✓ Bamboo shoots

✓ Rhubarb

✓ Bell pepper

✓ Rutabaga (swede)

✓ Bok choy

✓ Snow peas

✓ Broccoli

✓ Sprouts

✓ Brussels sprouts

✓ Sugar snap peas

✓ Cauliflower

✓ Summer squash

- ✓ Carrot

- ✓ Tomatoes

- ✓ Cucumber

- ✓ Turnip

- ✓ Celery

- ✓ Wax beans

- ✓ Green beans

- ✓ Water chestnuts

- ✓ Jicama

- ✓ Zucchini

- ✓ Mushrooms

Out of all the fibrous vegetables mentioned above, sugar snap peas, carrot and tomatoes are higher in sugar and therefore should be consumed in raw state only. Also, limit your consumption of these vegetables to ½ cup only.

Rule 4 – Eat recommended fats only.

The following is a list of fats that can be consumed on ketogenic diet. It is important to note that the diet emphasizes on consuming more saturated animal fats instead of vegetable oils. This helps with reducing the consumption of polyunsaturated fatty acids.

Fats that can be used for cooking:

✓ Butter– cook on low temperature. Look for organic sources

✓ Beef tallow – preferably from grass-fed sources

✓ Organic duck fat

✓ Organic chicken fat

✓ Ghee

✓ Olive oil (cold pressed, organic)

✓ Organic lard

✓ Organic coconut oil, coconut cream concentrate, and coconut butter

✓ Organic red palm oil

Fats for Cold Dressings:

✓ Macadamia oil

✓ Avocado oil

✓ Mayonnaise –is rich in soybean oil. Therefore, mayonnaise should be used in small amounts only. It is best to go with a homemade version.

✓ Seed and other nut oils –sesame oil, almond oil, flaxseed oil, etc. These oils are rich in omega 6 fats, so it is best to limit the amount and don't heat these oils.

✓ Avoid using vegetable oils as much as you can. These varieties include canola oil, corn oil, safflower oil, grapeseed oil, rice bran, sunflower oil, etc.) These oils are high in omega 6 fats and are inflammatory.

Rule 5 – The following foods fall into the "allowed" category but should only be consumed in limited quantities.

Cheese: can be consumed up to 4oz/day

- ✓ Keep a check of carb count, which should be less than 1g/serving.

- ✓ Aged, hard cheeses such as cheddar and Swiss cheese.

- ✓ Soft cheese such as goat, mozzarella, blue, camembert, brie cheese.

- ✓ Block and whipped cream cheese without any whey content.

- ✓ Avoid processed cheeses such as velveeta.

Dairy Cream: Can be consumed up to 4 tbsp/day

- ✓ Always check labels and do not eat any product that includes whey

- ✓ Avoid using mil or half-and-half. These are too many carbs.

- ✓ Heavy cream, sour cream, or whipping cream.

Fatty Vegetables

- ✓ Avocado. Limit the consumption to only ½avocado per day.

- ✓ Olives (both green and black versions allowed). Up to 7 olives can be consumed in a day.

Mayonnaise: Can be consumed up to 4 tbsp/day

- ✓ Always check labels for carb content.

- ✓ Less than 1 carb/serving.

Other Condiments

- ✓ Lime juice/lemon –4 tsp/day

- ✓ Ketchup – preferably homemade (low-sugar). Can be used 1 tbsp per day.

- ✓ Salad dressings – preferably homemade from vinegar and oil. Do not use balsamic vinegar. Spices and sour cream can be used.

- ✓ Soy sauces –4 tbsp per day.

- ✓ Pickles: check the labels for the right serving size and carb content.

  - – Sugar-free or dill

  - – Sugar-free pickles

- ✓ Stevia and spices or other artificial sweeteners in small portions.

Baking/Snacks

- ✓ Nut and nut flours in very small amounts. Restrict consumption to 1oz. per day

- ✓ Pork rinds

- ✓ Avoid snacks that include whey protein.

Allowed Beverages

✓ Clear bouillon or broth

✓ Almond milk (unsweetened) – limit consumption to 2 cups/day

✓ Decaf tea (unsweetened)

✓ Decaf coffee

✓ Herbal tea (unsweetened)

✓ Water

Follow these rules and keep a check on your shopping list before you begin. The next chapter includes some delicious, scrumptious recipes to make your ketogenic diet easy and fun.

The recipes are easy to follow and prepared with ketogenic diet rules in mind. Don't forget to mark your favorite ones to enjoy the diet throughout!

Chapter 3: Scrumptious Quick Recipes To Help You Get Started

Breakfast

Here are some interesting breakfast recipes to begin your day. Follow the steps and keep the nutritional information in mind to adjust your portions accordingly.

Savory Cheddar and Sage Waffles

Different from the regular waffles, these unique cheddar and sage waffles will make the perfect treat for breakfast time. The leftover waffles base can also be used for open-faced sandwiches for lunch or dinner time. Enjoy the complimenting flavors of sage and cheddar cheese and relish the recipe.

Nutritional Information (Per Serving)

- Calories 213.92

- Fats 17.21g

- Fiber 5.4g

- Net carbs3.81g

- Protein 6.52g

Serves: 6-8

Preparation Time: 10 minutes

Cooking Time: 10 minutes

Ingredients

- Coconut flour (sifted), 1 1/3 cup

- Salt, ½ tsp

- Baking powder, 3 tsp

- Ground sage (dried), 1 tsp

- Water, ½ cup

- Garlic powder, ¼ tsp

- Coconut milk (canned), 2 cups

- 2 Eggs

- Coconut oil (melted), 3 tbsp

- Cheddar cheese (shredded), 1 cup

Directions

1. Set your waffle iron to heat following the manufacturer's directions.

2. In a large mixing bowl, whisk all the dry ingredients together – including b baking powder, flour, and seasoning.

3. Add all the liquid ingredients to the dry mixture and stir until it forms a thick batter. Stir in cheese.

4. Grease the waffle iron once it is heated. Add scoop of batter onto each section of the iron. Close and cook until done.

5. Remove and transfer to a platter. Serve with avocado slices and maple syrup on the top. Enjoy!

Breakfast Tacos

Nutrition Information (Per Serving)

– Calories 443

– Fats 36.2g

– Fiber 1.7g

– Net carbs 3g

– Protein 25.7

Serves: 3

Preparation Time: 10 minutes

Cooking Time: 25 minutes

Ingredients

– 6 Large eggs

– 1 small avocado

– Butter, 2 tbsp

– Cheddar cheese (shredded), 1 oz.

– Bacon, 3 strips

– Salt, to taste

– Freshly ground black pepper, to taste

Directions

1. Place bacon strips on a lined baking sheet and bake at 375 degrees F for 15-20 minutes until done.

2. Meanwhile, heat 1/3 cup of mozzarella on a nonstick pan to prepare the shells.

3. Do not flip until the cheese turns brown on all sides. This will take 2-3 minutes.

4. Use tongs to lift up the cheese shell and drape it on a wooden spoon to give it the perfect taco shape. Follow the same method for the remaining cheese working in batches of 1/3 cups at a time.

5. Add butter to the pan and heat. Stir in eggs and cook until they are done. Season with salt and pepper.

6. Once the cheese taco shells are hardened, spoon avocado, scrambled eggs, and cooked bacon in each.

7. Sprinkle remaining cheddar cheese on the top.

8. Add fresh chopped cilantro and some hot sauce for additional flavor if you like.

9. Serve and enjoy!

Bacon and Cheddar Omelet

Nutrition Information (Per Serving)

- Calories 463

- Fats 39g

- Fiber 0g

- Net carbs 1g

- Protein 24g

Serves: 1

Preparation Time: 5 minutes

Cooking Time: 10 minutes

Ingredients

- Bacon fat, 1 tsp

- Bacon (cooked), 2 slices

- Cheddar cheese, 1 oz.

- 2 large eggs

- 2 stalks of chives

- Salt to taste

- Ground black pepper, to taste

Directions

1. Place a nonstick pan over low-med heat and add bacon fat. Stir in eggs and season with salt, pepper and chopped chives.

2. Let cook until the edges of the eggs starts to set. Add bacon on the center of the eggs and let cook for another 20 seconds. Turn off the stove.

3. Add cheese on top of the bacon and fold one side of the omelet like a burrito.

4. Press with a spoon and hold the other side until it is glued by the melting cheese.

5. Flip over to warm on the other side.

6. Serve with more chopped chives on the top and enjoy.

Pour Egg-Cups

Nutrition Information (Per Serving)

- Calories 215.8
- Fats 19.3g
- Fiber 0.2g
- Net carbs 0.9g
- Protein 9.6g

Serves: 12 muffins

Preparation Time: 10 minutes

Cooking Time: 25 minutes

Ingredients

- 12 bacon strips
- Cheddar cheese, 4 oz.
- 8 large eggs
- Cream cheese, 3 oz.
- Jalapeno pepper (deseeded and chopped), 4 medium peppers
- Onion powder, ½ tsp
- Garlic powder, ½ tsp
- Salt, to taste
- Ground black pepper, to taste

Directions

1. Set the oven to preheat setting at 375 degrees F. Par cook bacon strips so they are already semi-crispy but pliable. Save the grease from the bacon to add to the mixture.

2. Use a hand mixer to combine all ingredients (except cheddar cheese and 1 jalapeno pepper) together.

3. Grease the muffin tin and place the pre-cooked bacon strips around the edges.

4. Pour the mixture of eggs into the muffin tin. Do not over fill.

5. Garnish with cheddar cheese on top and place one jalapeno ring.

6. Set to bake for 20-25 minutes until done.

7. Remove from the oven and let cool. Serve on a large platter and adjust seasoning if required.

8. Enjoy!

Peanut Pancakes

Nutrition Information (Per Serving)

- Calories 539.1

- Fats 50.7g

- Fiber 5.1g

- Net carbs 6.2g

- Protein 16.1g

Serves: 2 muffins

Preparation Time: 10 minutes

Cooking Time: 5 minutes

Ingredients for Peanut Filling

- Fresh shelled peanuts, 1.8 oz.

- Stevia, ½ tsp

- Salt, to taste

Ingredients for Condensed Milk

- Heavy cream, ¼ cup

- Liquid sucralose, 2 drops

Ingredients for Apam Balik

- Almond flour, ½ cup

- Bicarbonate soda, ½ tsp

- Baking powder, ½ tsp

- Salt, 1/8 tsp

- Almond milk, ¼ cup

- 1 large egg

- Vanilla extract, ½ tsp

- Liquid sucralose, 4 drops

- Coconut oil, ¼ tsp

- Unsalted butter, 1 tbsp

Directions

1. Deshell peanuts and roast until brown. Grind with stevia and add salt as per your taste.

2. Heat a small saucepan and add heavy cream. Add a few drops of liquid sucralose until the mixture is thickened like condensed milk.

3. In a large mixing bowl, combine almond flour with baking powder, baking soda and some salt. Add in almond milk, liquid sucralose, egg, and vanilla extract. Mix well.

4. Heat a pan and add coconut oil. Stir in half of the pancake mixture like you will cook any other pancake. Cover the pan for a minute.

5. Sprinkle the sweetened ground peanuts on the pancakes and spread half of the condensed milk on top with some butter.

6. Cover and let cook for another minute.

7. Remove when done and repeat the method to cook another pancake.

8. Fold and serve.

<u>Bacon Devilled Hard-Boiled Eggs</u>

Nutrition Information (Per Serving)

– Calories 331

– Fats 30.3g

– Fiber 0g

– Net carbs 1.8g

– Protein 14.5g

Serves: 3

Preparation Time: 5 minutes

Cooking Time: 25 minutes

Ingredients

– Mayonnaise, ¼ cup

– 5 large eggs, hard boiled

– Cayenne pepper, ¼ tsp

– Bacon, 2 slices

– Rosemary, ½ tsp

– Dijon mustard, ¼ tsp

– Bacon fat (all fat rendered), 1 tbsp

Directions

1. Cut bacon into small and thin slices and place them in a nonstick pan over low-med heat. Stir occasionally as you cook bacon completely.

2. Remove bacon and transfer to a plate with paper towels. Reserve as much bacon drippings as you can in the pan. Let the cooked bacon cool down to become crispy.

3. Slice your hard boiled eggs into two. Remove eggs and reserve in a bowl.

4. Add Dijon mustard, mayonnaise, reserved bacon fat, cayenne pepper, and half of the rosemary in the yolk and mix until thoroughly incorporated. Reserve some rosemary for garnish.

5. Assemble eggs on a platter. Fill the yolk area with some bacon pieces and top with a spoon full of the yolk-mayonnaise mixture.

6. Top with remaining bacon and rosemary.

7. Serve for breakfast and enjoy.

Egg and Bacon Salad

Nutrition Information (Per Serving)

– Calories 344

– Fats 30.9g

– Fiber 0.24g

– Net carbs 2.1g

– Protein 15.5g

Serves: 3

Preparation Time: 10 minutes

Cooking Time: 20 minutes

Ingredients

– 4-5 large eggs, hard boiled

– Bacon, 3 slices

– Mayonnaise, ¼ cup

– Dijon mustard, 2 tsp

– ¼ tsp red onion (medium)

– Bacon fat, 2 tbsp

– Freshly grounded black pepper, ¼ tsp

– Cayenne pepper, ¼ tsp

Directions

1. Cut bacon into small pieces and place on a nonstick pan over low-med heat. Cook until done and crispy. Remove from pan and place on paper towels. Reserve drippings.

2. Meanwhile, slice the red onion. Add to the hard boiled eggs along with ¼ cup mayonnaise, 2 tbsp Dijon mustard, and bacon drippings.

3. Smash as you mix the ingredients until the mixture reaches its desired consistency.

4. Add spices and mix again.

5. Add bacon to the mix and gently fold in to keep it crispy and chunky.

6. Serve fresh for best flavors.

<u>Blueberry Crepes with Cream</u>

Nutrition Information (Per Serving)

- Calories 130

- Fats 10.6g

- Fiber 0.1g

- Net carbs 2.3g

- Protein 9.6g

Serves: 6 crepes

Preparation Time: 10 minutes

Cooking Time: 30 minutes

Ingredients for Crepes

- Cream cheese, 2 oz.

- Cinnamon, ¼ tsp

- 2 large eggs

- Baking soda, ¼ tsp

- Liquid stevia, 10 drops

- Sea salt, 1/8 tsp

- Coconut oil or butter, for greasing

Ingredients for Cream Filling

- Cream cheese, 4 oz.

- Blueberries, 60g

- Powdered erythritol, 2 tbs

- Vanilla extract, ½ tsp

Directions

1. To prepare the crepe batter, combine eggs and cream cheese in a mixing bowl using an electric hand mixer. Continue to blend until completely smooth.

2. Add cinnamon, stevia, sea salt, and baking soda to the mixture. Combine well.

3. Prepare a nonstick pan and place over low-med heat. Add some coconut oil or butter to grease lightly.

4. Pour in about ¼ cup of the batter into the pan. Swirl as you pour and spread equally from the edges. Cook for 2-3 minutes on both sides. Use a spatula to wiggle the edges and loosen them. Flip gently.

5. Continue with the remaining batter to prepare all six crepes.

6. Meanwhile, prepare the filling by mixing cream cheese with powdered erythritol and vanilla extract in a mixing bowl. Use a hand mixer to blend the ingredients until creamy and smooth.

7. When the crepes are ready, add some of the filling in the center of each crepe. Add fresh blueberries and wrap it up.

8. Sprinkle with cinnamon on top and serve fresh.

__Keto Bagel__

Nutrition Information (Per Serving)

- Calories 352

- Fats 19g

- Fiber 20g

- Net carbs 8g

- Protein 18g

Serves: 6 small bagels

Preparation Time: 20 minutes

Cooking Time: 55 minutes

Ingredients

- Psyllium fiber, ¼ cup

- Coconut flour, 1 cup

- Hemp hearts, ½ cup

- Sesame seeds, ½ cup

- Celtic sea, 1 tsp

- Pumpkin seeds, ½ cup

- 6 organic egg whites

- Baking powder, 1 tbsp

Directions

1. Set the oven to preheat setting at 350 degrees F.

2. Add all the dry ingredients to a large mixing bowl and stir to combine.

3. Add egg whites in a blender and blend until foamy. Stir into the dry ingredients mixture with a spoon. Fold to combine well.

4. The dough will be slightly crumbly after mixing.

5. Add 1 cup of boiling water to the dough and continue to stir until it forms a smoother batter/dough form.

6. After adding water, the dough will remain crumbly but will stick together when formed into a ball.

7. Prepare a cookie sheet and line with parchment paper.

8. Form six equal size balls from the dough. Press it down between your hands to give it a bagel shape and press in the center to create a little hole. Place the bagel on the cookie sheet.

9. Sprinkle with some poppy seeds or sesame seeds so it looks pretty.

10. Set to bake for about 55 minutes at the same temperature.

11. When done, turn off the heat but let the bagel sit in the oven for a few more minutes for a crunchier top.

12. Remove from oven and let the temperature settle.

13. Serve with your favorite Ketogenic filling and enjoy the delicious bagels for breakfast.

Raspberry Pudding

Nutrition Information (Per Serving)

- Calories 223

- Fats 18.2g

- Fiber 7.7g

- Net carbs 4.2g

- Protein 5.5g

Serves: 4

Preparation Time: 30 minutes

Cooking Time: --

Ingredients

- Coconut milk, 1 cup

- Frozen or fresh raspberries, 1 cup

- Water, ½ cup

- Chia seeds (whole) ½ cup

- Stevia to taste

- Vanilla powder, 1 tsp

Directions

1. Add water, coconut milk, and raspberries into a high immersion blender and pulse until all ingredients are blended. Reserve some raspberries for topping.

2. Pour the raspberry milk in a serving container and add chia seed. Mix to adjust the ingredients.

3. Add vanilla and sweetener as per your taste. Combine again to adjust flavors.

4. Refrigerate the mixture for 20-30 minutes. Spoon the prepared pudding into serving bowls.

5. Top with fresh raspberries and serve immediately for delicious flavors.

Main Course

Here are 22 main course recipes – including soups, salads and dips – that can be used for lunch and dinner. The leftovers can also be used for next day. Try out these recipes and don't forget to mark your favorite ones!

Avocado Chicken Sandwich

Nutrition Information (Per Serving)

- Calories 361
- Fats 28.2g
- Fiber 2g
- Net carbs 2g
- Protein 22g

Serves: 2

Preparation Time: 15 minutes

Cooking Time: 25 minutes

Ingredients for Cloud Bread

- 3 large eggs
- Cream of tartar, 1/8 tsp
- Cream cheese, 3 oz.
- Salt, 1/4tsp
- Garlic powder, ½ tsp

Ingredients for Filling

- Sriracha, 1 tsp

- Mayonnaise, 1 tbsp

- Bacon, 2 slices

- Chicken, 3 oz.

- Pepper jack cheese, 2 slices

- ¼ medium-sized avocado

- 2 Grape tomatoes

Directions

1. Set the oven to preheat setting at 300 degrees F.

2. Break the eggs and separate the yolks and place them in a different bowl.

3. Add salt and cream of tartar to the egg whites and whip until foamy and soft.

4. Add cream cheese to the yolks and beat until the mixture is well combined and forms pale yellow color.

5. Add the foamy egg white mixture into the yolk mixture and fold them well.

6. Prepare a baking sheet with parchment paper. Spoon ¼ of the batter on top and give it a square shape. Continue with the remaining batter. The four cloud bread will make two sandwiches.

7. Sprinkle garlic powder on top of each and set to bake for 25 minutes in a preheated oven.

8. Meanwhile, cook bacon and chicken in a nonstick pan with some salt and pepper.

9. Once the cloud bread is ready, assemble your sandwich with mayo, halved tomatoes, cooked chicken and bacon mixture, sriracha, mashed avocados, and cheese.

10. Serve immediately and enjoy.

Cheese-Stuffed Hot Dogs

Nutrition Information (Per Serving)

- Calories 379.7

- Fats 34.5g

- Fiber 0g

- Net carbs 0.3g

- Protein 16.8g

Serves: 6

Preparation Time: 10 minutes

Cooking Time: 40 minutes

Ingredients

- 6 hot dogs

- Cheddar cheese, 2 oz.

- Bacon, 12 slices

- Garlic powder, ½ tsp

- Onion powder, ½ tsp

- Salt, to taste

- Ground black pepper, to taste

Directions

1. Set the oven to preheat setting at 400 degrees F.

2. Carefully cut a slit in all the hot dogs and fill it up with cheese slices.

3. Wrap all the hot dogs in two slices of bacon and secure using toothpicks.

4. Once the hot dogs are ready, place them on top of a wire rack over a cookie sheet.

5. Season with salt and pepper as per your taste and set to bake for 35-40 minutes.

6. Serve hot and enjoy!

Green Bean Fries

Nutrition Information (Per Serving)

- Calories 113

- Fats 6.3g

- Fiber 0.2g

- Net carbs 2.4g

- Protein 9.3g

Serves: 4

Preparation Time: 10 minutes

Cooking Time: 10 minutes

Ingredients

- Green beans, 12 oz.

- 1 egg

- Parmesan cheese (grated), 2/3 cup

- Ground black pepper, ¼ tsp

- Pink Himalayan salt, ½ tsp

- Paprika, ¼ tsp

- Garlic powder, ½ tsp

Directions

1. Set the oven to preheat setting at 400 degrees F.

2. Wash and dry the green beans completely and make sure you chop the ends off.

3. In a small shallow plate, combine parmesan cheese with all the seasonings and combine well.

4. In a medium-sized bowl, whisk an egg. Make sure the bowl is big enough to place in beans.

5. Drench a handful of beans in the eggs and lift to drop off any excess. Now place the drenched beans into the parmesan mixture and roll to cover on all sides.

6. Place the coated beans on a greased baking sheet. Continue will the remaining beans and sprinkle the leftover cheese mixture on top.

7. Set to bake for 10 minutes until the beans turn slightly golden.

8. Remove from oven and let cool for a while. Serve with ranch or mayo dip and enjoy.

Note: This recipe can be used as a main course as well as a sideline.

Garlic Shrimp

Nutrition Information (Per Serving)

- Calories 335

- Fats 27g

- Fiber 0.1g

- Net carbs 2.5g

- Protein 22.3g

Serves: 2

Preparation Time: 5 minutes

Cooking Time: 5 minutes

Ingredients

- Large shrimp, ½lb

- Garlic, 3 cloves

- Olive oil, ¼ cup

- 1 lemon wedge

- Cayenne, ¼ tsp

- Salt, to taste

- Ground black pepper, to taste

Directions

1. Place a small nonstick pan over low-med heat and add olive oil. Stir in cayenne and minced garlic.

2. Let cook for a minute until the garlic is fragrant.

3. Peel and devein shrimp (if not done earlier). Add to the pan and stir to coat oil on all sides.

4. Cook for 3-4 minutes until pink.

5. Season with salt and pepper as per your preference and squeeze one lemon wedge into the pan.

6. Stir to adjust flavors and transfer to a platter.

7. Serve hot with garlic butter on the side as a dip.

<u>Steak and Eggs</u>

Nutrition Information (Per Serving)

– Calories 510

– Fats 36g

– Fiber 0.1g

– Net carbs 3g

– Protein 44g

Serves: 1

Preparation Time: 5 minutes

Cooking Time: 25 minutes

Ingredients

– Butter, 1 tbsp

– Sirloin, 4 oz.

– 3 eggs

– ¼ medium-sized avocado

– Salt, to taste

– Black pepper, to taste

Directions

1. Place a nonstick pan over low-med heat. Add butter and let it melt.

2. Add 2-3 eggs and fry until whites are completely set and yolk is desirably done. Season with salt and pepper as per your preference. Set aside.

3. In another pan, cook sirloin until it reaches your desired doneness. You can use any other cut of steak if you like.

4. Slice it done to bite-size strips once it is cool enough to handle. Season with salt and pepper.

5. In a platter, adjust the sirloin as a base layer and cover it up with some avocado chunks. Top with fried eggs and serve.

Note: The recipe can also be used as a delicious breakfast option if you like!

Egg Soup

Nutrition Information (Per Serving)

- Calories 276

- Fats 23g

- Fiber 0g

- Net carbs 2.5g

- Protein 12g

Serves: 1

Preparation Time: 5 minutes

Cooking Time: 20 minutes

Ingredients

- Chicken broth, 1 ½ cups

- Bacon fat (or any butter), 1 tbsp

- Chicken bouillon, ½ cube

- 2 large eggs

- Chili garlic paste, 1 tsp

Directions

1. Place a nonstick pan over med-high heat.

2. Add chicken broth, bacon fat, and bouillon cube. Stir well.

3. Bring the broth to a boil and stir in chili garlic paste. Stir well to adjust the flavors. Turn off the stove.

4. Beat eggs in a small bowl and add to the steamy broth. Stir immediately and create the swirls.

5. Cover and let sit for a moment before serving hot soup in bowls.

Pumpkin Carbonara

Nutrition Information (Per Serving)

- Calories 384

- Fats 34.7g

- Fiber 2g

- Net carbs 2g

- Protein 14g

Serves: 3

Preparation Time: 10 minutes

Cooking Time: 25 minutes

Ingredients

- Shirataki noodles, 1 pkg.

- 2 large eggs (yolks only)

- Pancetta, 5 oz.

- Heavy cream, ¼ cup

- Pumpkin puree, 3 tbsp

- Butter, 2 tbsp

- Dried sage, ½ tsp

- Pumpkin puree, 3 tbsp

- Salt, to taste

- Black pepper, to taste

Directions

1. Prepare shirataki noodles as per the instructions on the package. When done, dry them completely and set aside.

2. Place a pan over low-med heat. Add chopped pancetta into the pan and sear on the outside. Once it is done, remove and set aside, reserving the fats in the pan.

3. In another small pot, add butter and place it over low-med heat. When the butter melts down and starts to brown, add in pumpkin puree and sage. Add reserved pancetta fat and heavy cream to the pot and mix well.

4. Reheat the pan that had pancetta fat and add shirataki noodles and adjust the flame to high. Fry dry for 5 minutes until it becomes steamy.

5. Meanwhile, add parmesan cheese to the pumpkin puree mixture and combine well. Adjust heat to low and simmer until it becomes thick.

6. Add fried noodles to the pot along with pancetta to the pumpkin sauce and toss to combine.

7. Add 2 egg yolks and stir continuously until it is mixed well.

8. Serve hot and enjoy.

Kung Pao Chicken

Nutrition Information (Per Serving)

– Calories 361.7

– Fats 27.4g

– Fiber 1.3g

– Net carbs 3.2g

– Protein 22.3g

Serves: 3

Preparation Time: 5 minutes

Cooking Time: 25 minutes

Ingredients

– 2 medium chicken thigh (with skin and bone)

– Peanuts, ¼ cup

– Ground ginger, 1 tsp

– Salt, to taste

– Ground black pepper, to taste

– 2 large spring onions, chopped

– 4 Red Bird's Eye chili, de-seeded

– ½ medium green-pepper

Ingredients for Sauce

- Soy sauce, 1 tbsp

- Chili garlic paste, 2 tbsp

- Rice wine vinegar, 2 tsp

- Ketchup (preferably homemade or reduced sugar), 1 tbsp

- Sesame oil, 2 tsp

- Liquid stevia, 10 drops

- Maple extract, ½ tsp

Directions

1. Chop chicken to small, bite-size pieces and season with ginger, salt, and pepper.

2. Place a pan over med-high heat and add chicken. Cook for 8-10 minutes until brown on all sides.

3. Chop all the vegetables and set aside.

4. Add all the ingredients to prepare sauce and whisk together in a small bowl until combined well. Set aside.

5. When chicken is cooked, stir in all the remaining ingredients (except sauce). Stir to combine. Cook for another few minutes until everything is heated through.

6. Add peanuts and vegetables in the pan and cook for 3-4 minutes.

7. Add sauce and stir again to combine. Adjust seasoning if you like.

8. Bring the mixture to a boil to reduce and thicken the texture.

9. Serve hot.

Keto Pizza

Nutrition Information (Per Serving)

- Calories 459
- Fats 35g
- Fiber 8.5g
- Net carbs 3.5g
- Protein 27g

Serves: 1

Preparation Time: 10 minutes

Cooking Time: 20 minutes

Ingredients for Crust

- 2-3 eggs
- Psyllium husk powder, 1 tbsp
- Parmesan cheese, 2 tbsp
- Italian seasoning, ½ tsp
- Frying oil (use butter or bacon fat), 2 tsp
- Salt, to taste

Ingredients for Toppings

- Mozzarella cheese, 1.5 oz.
- Rao's tomato sauce, 3 tbsp
- Basil (Freshly chopped), 1 tbsp

Directions

1. Place all the pizza crust ingredients in an immersion blender container and blend at high speed to mix well.

2. Place a nonstick frying pan over low-med heat and spread out the crust mixture in a large circle.

3. Cook for a few minutes until the edges start to set. Flip and cook for another minute. Turn off the flame.

4. Turn on the broiler to preheat.

5. Spread tomato sauce and cheese on the crust. Cover with cheese.

6. Set to broil for 1-2 minutes until the cheese starts to melt and begins bubbling.

7. Remove from the oven and serve hot.

Ginger Glazed Salmon

Nutrition Information (Per Serving)

– Calories 370

– Fats 23.5g

– Fiber 0g

– Net carbs 2.5g

– Protein 33g

Serves: 2

Preparation Time: 20 minutes

Cooking Time: 25 minutes

Ingredients

– Salmon fillet, 10 oz.

– Sesame oil, 2 tsp

– Soy sauce (or coconut aminos), 2 tbsp

– Rice vinegar, 1 tbsp

– Garlic (minced),2 tsp

– Ginger (minced), 1 tsp

– Ketchup (sugarfree), 1 tbsp

– Red boat fish sauce, 1 tbsp

– White wine, 2 tbsp

Directions

1. Add all the ingredients along with fish fillet (except for white wine, ketchup and sesame oil) in a Tupperware container.

2. Let the fish fillet soak in the liquid ingredients for 10-15 minutes.

3. Place a nonstick pan over med-high heat and add sesame oil. Adjust heat to low-med once the pan is hot. Add fish fillet (skin down) to the pan carefully

4. Place all the pieces and let cook for 3-4 minutes until the skin looks crisp. Flip and cook on the other side for another 2-3 minutes.

5. Add the marinate liquids over the fillet and let that cook while the fillets are cooking. The liquids will boil and reduce, leaving a glazed-like texture.

6. When fish is cooked, remove from the pan and transfer to a serving platter. Reserve the glazed liquids in the pan and place it back on the heat.

7. Add ketchup and white wine to the mixture in the pan and stir to combine. Simmer for 5 minutes over low-med heat until the mixture reduces.

8. Drizzle on top of the fillets and serve hot for delicious flavors.

Lemon Shrimp Pasta

Nutrition Information (Per Serving)

- Calories 360

- Fats 21g

- Fiber 0.3g

- Net carbs 3.5g

- Protein 36g

Serves: 4

Preparation Time: 10 minutes

Cooking Time: 10 minutes

Ingredients

- Angel hair noodle, 2 pkg.

- 4 garlic cloves

- Olive oil, 2 tbsp

- Butter, 2 tbsp

- ½ lemon

- Paprika, ½ tsp

- Large raw shrimp, 1 lb

- Fresh basil

- Salt, to taste

- Ground black pepper, to taste

Directions

1. Prepare noodles as per the instructions on the package. When cooked, rinse through cold water, drain, and transfer to a nonstick pan.

2. Place the pan over low-med heat and dry roast them to evaporate moisture completely. When noodles are dried out completely, remove and set aside.

3. Add butter in the same pan along with olive oil and let heat. Crush garlic and add to the pan and cook for a minute until fragrant.

4. Cut lemon into thin slices. Add shrimp to the pan along with lemon slices. Stir and cook for 2-3 minutes. Flip sides to make sure shrimps are cooked on all sides.

5. When the shrimp are opaque and cooked, add noodles and mix well. Adjust flavors and season with salt, paprika, and pepper. Mix again.

6. Toss everything so flavors are well combined.

7. Sprinkle chopped fresh basil on top and transfer to a serving plate. Enjoy!

<u>Cob Salad</u>

Nutrition Information (Per Serving)

– Calories 600

– Fats 48g

– Fiber 3g

– Net carbs 3g

– Protein 43g

Serves: 1-2

Preparation Time: 10 minutes

Cooking Time: --

Ingredients

– Spinach, 1 cup

– Bacon, 2 strips

– 1 large egg, hard boiled

– Chicken breast, 2 oz

– ¼ Avocado

– ½ campari tomato

– Olive oil, 1 tbsp

– White vinegar, ½ tsp

Directions

1. Prepare your chicken and bacon as per your preference. It is best to use leftover chicken or bacon or pre-cooked ones to prepare this salad. Slice the chicken in small chunks.

2. Chop all ingredients into small pieces.

3. Combine vegetables, bacon, and chicken together. Add vinegar and oil and toss to adjust flavors.

4. Toss well and serve.

Crack Slaw

Nutrition Information (Per Serving)

- Calories 350

- Fats 27g

- Fiber 2g

- Net carbs 4g

- Protein 24g

Serves: 4

Preparation Time: 10 minutes

Cooking Time: 15 minutes

Ingredients

- Sesame seed oil, 2 tbsp

- Garlic, 2 cloves

- Lean ground beef, 1 lb

- Srirarcha, 1 tbsp

- Cole slaw salad mix, 10 oz

- Vinegar, 1 tsp

- Soy sauce, 2 tbsp

- Black pepper, ¼ tsp

- Sesame seeds, ½ tsp

- Pink Himalayan sea salt, ½ tsp

- 1 stalk green onion

Directions

1. Place a large wok over med-high heat and add sesame seed oil in it. Add crushed garlic and cook for a minute until it's fragrant.

2. Stir in ground beef and break using a spatula as you start cooking it. Mix well.

3. Continue stirring and cooking for 5-10 minutes until the ground beef is thoroughly browned on all sides. Add cole slaw salad mix to the wok and toss to combine all ingredients.

4. Stir in sriracha, vinegar, and soy sauce. Toss again to adjust flavors. Let the ingredients cook for another 5 minutes until everything is well incorporated and the claw slaw begins to wilt.

5. Season with sesame seeds, salt, and pepper. Serve with a sprinkle of fresh, chopped green onions. Serve and enjoy!

Cheddar Soup

Nutrition Information (Per Serving)

- Calories 370

- Fats 32g

- Fiber 1g

- Net carbs 8g

- Protein 11g

Serves: 4

Preparation Time: 10 minutes

Cooking Time: 40 minutes

Ingredients

- Butter, 1 tbsp

- Heavy cream, 1 cup

- ½ white onion (medium)

- Water, 2 cups

- Broth, 2 cups

- Broccoli, 12 oz.

- Salt, to taste

- Ground black pepper, to taste

- Cheddar, 8 oz.

- Paprika, ½ tsp

- Xantham gum, ¼ tsp

Directions

1. Place a large soup pot over low-med heat and add butter. Stir in onions and garlic and cook until onions are translucent and garlic is fragrant.

2. Stir in broth (you can use vegetable, chicken, or beef broth) along with cream and water to the pot. Stir to combine the ingredients and bring the mixture to a gentle boil.

3. Season with salt, pepper and paprika.

4. While the mixture is boiling, stir in fresh broccoli florets. This should be around four to six of florets. Stir to combine and adjust heat to low and let the soup simmer.

5. Cook broccoli for 25 minutes.

6. Once the broccoli is cooked, stir in cheddar and continue to cook. Allow the cheese to melt down completely. therefore, it is best to use shredded cheese as it will melt faster.

7. Turn off the stove after the cheese has melted completely. Allow the soup to cool down a bit and blend it after transferring it into an immersion blender. Continue until thoroughly smooth.

8. You can even use a hand blender to blend the smooth within the soup pot. Continue until the mixture is smooth and thick.

9. While you are blending the soup, stir in ¼ tsp of xanthan gum little after little. This will further improve the consistency of your soup and it will become thicker.

10. Sprinkle some more shredded cheddar cheese on top and heat the soup thoroughly before serving.

11. Dig in and enjoy!

Italian Casserole with Chicken and Cauliflower

Nutrition Information (Per Serving)

- Calories 300

- Fats 21g

- Fiber 3g

- Net carbs 2.5g

- Protein 29g

Serves: 6

Preparation Time: 20 minutes

Cooking Time: 20 minutes

Ingredients

- Olive oil, 1 tbsp

- Mushrooms, 2.5 oz.

- Chicken breast, 20 oz.

- Mayonnaise, ¼ cup

- Heavy cream, ¼ cup

- Cauliflower (riced), 2 cups

- Chicken stock, 1 cup

- Mozzarella cheese (shredded), ½ cup

- Low-carb vodka sauce, ½ cup

- Pork rinds, 1 oz.

- Parmesan cheese, 2 tbsp

- Salt, to taste

- Ground black pepper, to taste

- Garlic powder, to taste

- Oregano, for topping

Directions

1. Set the oven to preheat setting at 375 degrees F.

2. Start with ricing cauliflower until you are left with two-cup worth and cook in a pot with a cup of boiling broth for 10 minutes. You must ensure that the liquid from the broth evaporates completely.

3. At the same time, add chicken breasts to a pan and cook it.

4. Once the chicken is fully cooked, shred it. You can use two forks to help you shred the chicken in small chunks.

5. Stir in ¼ cup of heavy cream to the cooked cauliflower and continue cooking for another 5 minutes.

6. Slice mushrooms and add to the shredded chicken. Stir in ¼ cup mayonnaise and stir to combine everything.

7. Add in the creamy cauliflower to the bowl and stir well. Season to adjust flavors. You can use salt, oregano, pepper, and garlic powder for seasoning.

8. Stir in vodka sauce and continue to mix the ingredients.

9. Transfer the mixture into a baking dish and use a spatula to even it on the top.

10. Sprinkle shredded mozzarella cheese on top along with crushed pork rinds and parmesan.

11. Set to bake for 20 minutes. Check once midway to see if the dish is bubbling.

12. Garnish with fresh basil and serve immediately for best flavors.

Keto Guacamole

Nutrition Information (Per 2 tablespoon)

- Calories 77

- Fats 7g

- Fiber 0.01g

- Net carbs 1g

- Protein 1g

Serves: 1.5 cups

Preparation Time: 15 minutes

Cooking Time: --

Ingredients

- 2 ripe avocados

- 6 grape tomatoes

- Onions (diced), ¼ cup

- Garlic, 2 cloves

- ½ lime

- Olive oil, 1 tbsp

- Black pepper, 1/8 tsp

- Salt, ¼ tsp

- Cilantro (fresh), chopped

- Parsley (fresh), chopped

- Crushed red pepper, 1/8 tsp

Directions

1. Cut, pit and mash avocados in a large mixing bowl.

2. Dice tomatoes and onions and add them to the avocado mixture.

3. Squeeze garlic cloves and add to the mixture.

4. Add seasoning along with cilantro and parsley and mix to combine well.

5. Stir in lime juice and olive oil and whisk to mix.

6. Serve with low carb crackers or pork rinds.

7. Enjoy!

Mushroom Skewers

Nutrition Information (Per 2 skewers)

- Calories 110

- Fats 7g

- Fiber 0.02g

- Net carbs 2g

- Protein 9g

Serves: 6 skewers

Preparation Time: 15 minutes

Cooking Time: 20 minutes

Ingredients

- Bacon, 6 strips

- Sweet mesquite

- Mushrooms, 1 lb

- Skewers

Directions

1. Cut mushrooms in small pieces. Make sure the pieces aren't too small or they will fall through the grill gaps. They should be 'bite size'.

2. Place your skewers in water and soak them before threading the ingredients. This will keep them from catching fire during grilling. This method is only for wooden skewers.

3. Spear a bacon strip on the end of one skewer. Spear a mushroom and fold over the bacon strip, covering the entire mushroom pieces. Spear on the other end to wrap and tie.

4. Continue with the remaining skewers.

5. Season with sweet mesquite.

6. Set to grill for 15-20 minutes, flipping on the other side halfway through grilling. You can also bake them in the oven but grilling over charcoal guarantees best taste.

7. When done, serve on a platter and season more if you like. Enjoy!

Roasted Brussels Sprouts

Nutrition Information (Per serving)

– Calories 278

– Fats 21g

– Fiber 0g

– Net carbs 4g

– Protein 15g

Serves: 4

Preparation Time: 5 minutes

Cooking Time: 30 minutes

Ingredients

– Brussels sprouts, 1 lb

– Olive oil, 2 tbsp

– Bacon, 8 strips

– Salt, to taste

– Ground black pepper, to taste

Directions

1. Set the oven to preheat setting at 375 degrees F.

2. Cut the Brussels sprouts at the end and eliminate all the hard part. Then slice the sprouts in half or in quarters if they are too big in size.

3. Place the sliced Brussels sprouts in a large mixing bowl and drizzle with olive oil. Season with salt and pepper and toss well. Add any other spice if you like. Cumin and red pepper are some good options if you want to add some good flavor.

4. Grease a baking sheet and transfer the seasoned Brussels sprouts in it. Keep the sprouts in a single layer and with some space between them. Not all of them need to be on the same side.

5. Set to bake for 30 minutes. Half way through the baking time, remove carefully from the oven and shake well for a good rotation. Set it back until it is done.

6. Meanwhile, fry some bacon in a nonstick frying pan. You can use eight bacon strips (to feed four persons). When bacon is done cooking, remove and let cool. Chop it up in small pieces.

7. When sprouts are done, remove from own and transfer to a mixing bowl. Add chopped bacon and toss it up to combine well.

8. Serve on a platter and season with some more salt if needed. Serve and enjoy!

<u>Jalapeno Peppers wrapped in Bacon</u>

Nutrition Information (Per 4 Jalapenos)

- Calories 225

- Fats 17.9g

- Fiber 0.1g

- Net carbs 3.3g

- Protein 10.2g

Serves: 4 servings

Preparation Time: 20 minutes

Cooking Time: 20 minutes

Ingredients

- 16 Fresh jalapenos

- Cream cheese, 4 oz.

- 16 strips bacon

- Salt, 1 tsp

- Paprika, 1 tsp

- Cheddar cheese (shredded), ¼ cup

Direction

1. Set the oven to preheat setting at 350 degrees F.

2. Separate all the slices of bacon and cut them from center to create two slices from each and set aside. Slice the end of each jalapeno pepper and then cut it in half lengthwise. Remove membranes and seeds using a knife or corer. It is best to wear gloves to keep your hands protected.

3. Mix cheddar cheese and cream cheese together in a mixing bowl.

4. Fill each half of the jalapeno with this cream-cheese mixture.

5. Cover each half with bacon slice and place the wrapped poppers on a lined baking sheet. When all poppers are done, set to bake for 20-25 minutes until the jalapenos and bacon is baked completely.

6. You might want to do a taste test to make sure they are cooked according to your desired spiciness. The longer you cook jalapenos, the less spicy they are. You might want to cook a little longer so taste before you remove them from oven.

7. Season with salt, paprika and any other spice you like before serving.

8. Enjoy!

<u>One Pan Vegetable and Chicken Thighs</u>

Nutrition Information (Per serving)

- Calories 375

- Fats 32g

- Fiber 0g

- Net carbs 2g

- Protein 22g

Serves: 4 servings

Preparation Time: 15 minutes

Cooking Time: 30 minutes

Ingredients

- 4 Chicken thighs (skin on, deboned)

- Carrots (sliced), ½ cup

- 2 zucchinis

- Olive oil, ¼ cup

- Daikon radish, 1 cup

- Balsamic vinegar, 2 tbsp

- Ginger (minced), 1" cube

Directions

1. Set the oven to preheat setting at 350 degrees F. De-bone the chicken thighs and pat them dry. Let the skin on.

2. Wrap the skin around the thigh and arrange them on a baking sheet. Make sure the baking sheet is greased with butter or coconut oil beforehand.

3. Slice vegetables and arrange them around chicken in the baking sheet.

4. Whisk balsamic vinegar, olive oil, and minced ginger to make a sauce. Pour this mixture over the vegetables and chicken in the baking dish. Season with salt and pepper and set to bake for 30 minutes until chicken is completely cooked.

5. If you like your chicken crispy broil for 3-5 minutes more. Keep an eye on to avoid it from burning.

6. Serve and enjoy!

<u>Thai Beef Stir Fry</u>

Nutrition Information (Per serving)

- Calories 620

- Fats 43g

- Fiber 2g

- Net carbs 8g

- Protein 50g

Serves: 2 servings

Preparation Time: 20 minutes

Cooking Time: 20 minutes

Ingredients

- Garlic, 2 cloves

- Toasted sesame seed oil, 2 tbsp

- Ginger, 1 tsp

- ¼ red onion, medium

- 1 carrot

- 1 jalapeno

- 1 zucchini

- Lean beef, 1 lb

- Salt, ½ tsp

- Ground black pepper, ¼ tsp

- Chinese 5 spice, ¼ tsp

- Red pepper flakes, ¼ tsp

- Beef broth, ¼ cup

- Fresh basil (fresh), 1 bunch

- Cashews, 1 oz.

Directions

1. To make the cooking easier, chop all the veggies beforehand. Mince ginger and set aside. Slice jalapenos and carrots and leave the zucchini and onion a little chunky.

2. Add sesame seed oil in a wok over med-high heat. Stir in garlic, ginger, onion, and carrots. Stir and cook until onions are translucent and garlic is fragrant.

3. Add jalapenos and zucchini next along with the seasoning. Toss all the vegetables and combine well. Remove from the wok and set aside.

4. Stir in the thin slices of beef in the same wok. Add another tablespoon of sesame seed oil. Cook for 5-8 minutes until the beef strips are brown on all sides.

5. Add back vegetables and toss with the beef to combine. Add beef broth in the wok along with ¼ cup of coconut milk. You can even add heavy cream in place of coconut milk if you like.

6. Stir in cashews and continue cooking. Cover and cook for 8-10 minutes.

7. Last but not the least, add fresh basil leaves and stir to accommodate.

8. Cook for another 5 minutes and serve hot for delicious flavors.

Lemon and Mustard Pork

Nutrition Information (Per serving)

- Calories 480

- Fats 30g

- Fiber 1g

- Net carbs 1g

- Protein 46g

Serves: 2 servings

Preparation Time: 15 minutes

Cooking Time: 10 minutes

Ingredients for Pork Loins

- 4 pork loins, 4oz

- Thyme, 1 tsp

- Paprika, 1 tsp

- Black pepper, 1 tsp

- Pink Himalayan sea salt, 1 tbsp

Ingredients for Mustard Sauce

- Heavy cream, ¼ cup

- Chicken broth, ½ cup

- ½ lemon

- 1 tsp apple cider vinegar

- Mustard, 1 tbsp

Directions

1. Pat dry pork loins using a paper towel. Season with salt, paprika, pepper, and thyme.

2. Place a large nonstick pan over med-high heat. Place seasoned pork loins and sear on high heat on both sides for 2-3 minutes. When done, remove and set aside while you prepare the sauce.

3. Deglaze your pan with apple cider vinegar and chicken broth. Add ¼ cup of heavy cream and mix everything together. Adjust heat to low and let the mixture simmer for a few minutes.

4. Add lemon juice and 1 tablespoon mustard in the mixture. Stir and mix well.

5. Add seared pork loins in the sauce and cook. Flip once to coat with the sauce.

6. Let the pork loins cook for another 10 minutes with the lid of the pan slightly open.

7. When heated through, remove and transfer to a serving plate with sauce on top. Serve and enjoy!

Snacks

Ketogenic diet does not restrict you from enjoying snacks when you crave for them. While the food itself is quite filling and will not make you feel hungry for long, here are some interesting snack recipes to try if you are not in the mood for preparing a main-course meal for the day. If you just want to satisfy your cravings without cheating on your diet, check these recipes out!

Lemon Raspberry Popsicles

Nutrition Information (Per Serving)

- Calories 150.5

- Fats 16g

- Fiber 3.3g

- Net carbs 2g

- Protein 0.5g

Serves: 6

Preparation Time: 2 hours 10 minutes

Cooking Time: - -

Ingredients

- Raspberries, 100g

- Coconut oil, ¼ cup

- Juice of ½lemon

- Coconut milk, 1 cup

- Heavy cream, ¼ cup

- Sour cream, ¼ cup

- Liquid stevia, 20 drops

- Guar gum, ½ tsp

Directions

1. Place all the ingredients including the berries into the immersion blender container and blend it out.

2. Strain the mixture to separate the berry seeds and discard them.

3. Prepare the molds and carefully pour the mixture for popsicles. Set to freeze for at least 2 hours.

4. To serve, run the molds under warm water to dislodge the popsicle.

5. The berrilicious popsicles are ready to be served and enjoyed!

__Peanut Butter Chocolate Bombs__

Nutrition Information (Per Serving)

– Calories 208.3

– Fats 20g

– Fiber 2.4g

– Net carbs 0.8g

– Protein 4.4g

Serves: 8

Preparation Time: 30 minutes

Cooking Time: - -

Ingredients

– Coconut oil, ½ cup

– PB fit powder, 4 tbsp

– Cocoa powder, ¼ cup

– Shelled hemp seeds, 6 tbsp

– Vanilla extract, 1 tsp

– Heavy cream, 2 tbsp

– Liquid stevia, 28 drops

– Shredded coconut (unsweetened), ¼ cup

Directions

1. In a mixing bowl, add all the dry ingredients and sift to mix well. Add coconut oil and fold the ingredients until they become of a slightly wet consistency. Work it out until it forms a paste-like texture.

2. Add liquid stevia, vanilla, and heavy cream. Mix until everything is well combined and creamy.

3. In a flat plate, add shredded coconut.

4. Use the creamy paste to form balls with your hands and roll them in the shredded coconut to cover on all sides.

5. Lay on a prepared baking tray covered with parchment paper.

6. Set in the freezer for 20 minutes until done.

7. Serve chilled delicious chocolate bombs.

Pecan Bars

Nutrition Information (Per Serving)

- Calories 302.6

- Fats 30.5g

- Fiber 4.5g

- Net carbs 2g

- Protein 4.9g

Serves: 12

Preparation Time: 10 minutes

Cooking Time: 35-37 minutes

Ingredients

- Pecan halves, 2 cups

- Golden flaxseed meal, ½ cup

- Almond flour, 1 cup

- Shredded coconut (unsweetened), ½ cup

- Maple syrup, ¼ cup

- Coconut oil, ½ cup

- Liquid stevia, ¼ tsp

Directions

1. Set oven to preheat setting at 350 degrees F. Add pecans to a baking sheet and toast in the oven for 5-7 minutes. Remove and let cool.

2. Transfer roasted pecans in a plastic bag with seal. Crush using a rolling pin and set aside.

3. In a bowl, combine all dry ingredients. Stir in crushed pecans and mix well.

4. Add all the wet ingredients and mix again until it makes a dough-like texture. Transfer the dough in a large casserole dish and press it down to smooth out the surface.

5. Set to bake for 20-25 minutes at 350 degrees F.

6. When done, remove and place on a wire rack until completely cooled.

7. Set to refrigerate for another hour.

8. Cut into bar-like slices and serve.

Note: the bars can also be stored in an airtight container for 5 days.

Avocado Lime Sorbet

Nutrition Information (Per Serving)

– Calories 180

– Fats 18g

– Fiber 7.25g

– Net carbs 3.3g

– Protein 2g

Serves: 4

Preparation Time: 3 hours 20 minutes

Cooking Time: 20 minutes

Ingredients

– 2 medium-sized avocados

– Stevia, ¼ tsp

– Coconut milk, 1 cup

– Juice of 2 medium limes

– Zest of 2 medium limes

– Organic erythritol(powdered), ¼ cup

– Cilantro (chopped) ¼ cup

– Sliced avocados (optional)

Directions

1. Cut avocados into half and make thin slices. Scrape out the avocados completely. Place the scraped avocados and slices on a foil and squeeze juice from ½ lime.

2. Place it in the freezer for at least 3 hours. This can be done earlier before you are ready to prepare the snack.

3. Mix coconut milk, zest of 2 limes and powdered erythritol in a saucepan and bring the mixture to a gentle boil over med-high heat.

4. Allow the mixture to reduce by 25% and thicken. Pour it into a container and set to freeze until thickens.

5. Remove avocado from the freezer and place it into a food processor container. Add chopped cilantro and juice of 1 ½ limes. Pulse to puree the mixture. Continue until the processor is chunky. Add stevia and coconut milk mixture.

6. Grind until the mixture achieves desired consistency.

7. Serve with your favorite condiments or avocado slices on the side.

Coconut Cream Yogurt

Nutrition Information (Per Serving)

- Calories 314.5

- Fats 31.3g

- Fiber 0.3g

- Net carbs 4.3g

- Protein 0g

Serves: 4

Preparation Time: 20 minutes (Probiotic time can vary up to 24 days)

Cooking Time: - -

Ingredients

- Coconut milk (full fat), 1 can

- Xanthan gm, ½ tsp

- Organic probiotic-10, 2 capsules

- Heavy whipping cream, 2/3 cup

- Toppings, your choice

Directions

1. Open coconut milk can and stir well.

2. Empty it into a container. Add content of probiotic capsules into the container and place it in the oven light for 12-24 hours. This will allow you to collect maximum cream from the coconut milk. Do not open the oven before 12 hours. The longer you keep it, the more cream you can extract.

3. Once it is done, refrigerate it or place it directly into a mixing bowl.

4. Add xanthan gum to the yogurt and beat with a hand blender until well combined. The yogurt will thicken.

5. In a separate bowl, add heavy cream and whip until foamy. The consistency should be very stiff.

6. Add cream to yogurt and mix on speed. Combine all the ingredients and top with your favorite toppings.

7. Serve immediately or chill before serving and enjoy!

Beverages

You can't go wrong with the beverages when you are following ketogenic diet. And you have even a bit of doubt here, these recipes will keep you on track.

Strawberry Lemonade

Nutrition Information (Per Serving)

– Calories 96.7

– Fats 0.1g

– Fiber 0.73g

– Net carbs .2g

– Protein 0.04g

Serves: 4

Preparation Time: 15 minutes

Cooking Time: - -

Ingredients

– Frozen mixed berries, 1 cup

– Fresh mint, 1 cup

– 1 lime, cut into thin wedges

– 15-20 drops liquid stevia

– 1 bottle of sparkling water, 4 cups

– Ice

Directions

1. Wash mint and roughly chop it. Cut lime into thin wedge slices. Your mixed berry bowl can comprise of blackberries, wild blueberries, strawberries, raspberries, currants, and sour cherries.

2. Add all the ingredients in a large bottle and fill it up with 4 cups water.

3. Add stevia and shake the bottle once.

4. Leave it for 15 minutes or longer. You can refrigerate it and leave it for longer to get maximum flavors.

5. Add ice and enjoy.

Note: it is best to remove the peel of lime before putting them in your lemonade. This will keep your lemonade from getting bitter.

Mint Protein Shake

Nutrition Information (Per Serving)

– Calories 37

– Fats 2g

– Fiber 0g

– Net carbs 0.2g

– Protein 1g

Serves: 2

Preparation Time: 5 minutes

Cooking Time: - -

Ingredients

– Kale leaves, a handful

– Water, 1/3 cup

– Hemp seeds, 2 tbsp

– Egg-white protein powder, 1 scoop

– Vanilla stevia, 10 drops

– Peppermint extract, ¼ tsp

– Ice cubes, 1 cup

– Coconut oil, 1 tbsp

– Chocolate chips, 1 tbsp

Directions

1. Place protein powder, water, hemp seeds, and kale in a blender.

2. Pulse at high speed for 1-2 minutes until everything blends down and becomes smooth.

3. If your shake is too thick, add some more water to adjust consistency.

4. Add stevia, peppermint, and coconut oil in the mixture and blend again.

5. Add ice and blend once more.

6. When the shake is ready, add chocolate chips on top and serve chilled for delicious flavors.

Power Detox Smoothie

Nutrition Information (Per Serving)

- Calories 103.3

- Fats 1g

- Fiber 0.2g

- Net carbs 0.02g

- Protein 0.8g

Serves: 2

Preparation Time: 5 minutes

Cooking Time: - -

Ingredients

- Water or non-dairy milk, 1 cup

- 1 ripe banana

- Red cabbage, ½ cup

- Blueberries, ½ cup

- Kale leaves (chopped), 2 leaves

Directions

1. Add water or milk to the blender with all the remaining ingredients.

2. Pulse to mix and puree the ingredients until smooth. Use a high-immersion blender to get the perfect consistency so that it doesn't require straining.

3. Adjust flavors by adding some stevia or maple syrup if you like your smoothie sweet.

4. If the banana is ripe and sweet enough, you will not require any more sweetener.

5. Add ice and let sit for a bit. Serve in two glasses and enjoy.

Ice Tea

Nutrition Information (Per Serving)

– Calories 84

– Fats 0.02g

– Fiber 0.3g

– Net carbs 0g

– Protein 0.2g

Serves: 2

Preparation Time: 15 minutes

Cooking Time: 10 minutes

Ingredients

– Loose rooibos, 2 tbsp

– Almond extract, 1/8 tsp

– Boiling water, 2 cups

– Ice cubes, 2 cups

– 12 drops of stevia

– Coconut milk (full fat), ½ cup

Directions

1. Place loose rooibos tea in a 2-cup measuring container.

2. Add boiling water to the container along with stevia and almond extract.

3. Let sit for 15 minutes.

4. In two serving glasses, place ice cubes and strain the hot tea directly into the glasses.

5. Stir in some coconut milk and serve immediately for refreshing flavors.

Ginger Mocktail

Nutrition Information (Per Serving)

- Calories 120

- Fats 1.2g

- Fiber 0g

- Net carbs 0.01g

- Protein 0.3g

Serves: 2

Preparation Time: 5 minutes

Cooking Time: - -

Ingredients

- Freshly squeezed lime juice, ¼ cup

- Stevia, 12 drops

- Zested ginger, 1 tsp

- Sparkling water, 18 oz.

Directions

1. In a large jar, add all ingredients and shake well.

2. Add ice to two cocktail glasses and pour the mocktail in each glass.

3. Garnish with lime wedges and serve chilled for best flavors.

Desserts

Omitting sugar from your diet does not really mean you should give up desserts. After all, your sweet tooth needs to be taken care of from time to time. Keep a check on your portion size and try out these interesting, ketogenic-friendly dessert recipes!

Cheesecake Pumpkin Bars

Nutrition Information (Per Serving)

- Calories 159

- Fats 14g

- Fiber 5g

- Net carbs 3g

- Protein 3g

Serves: 16 bars

Preparation Time: 3 hours 30 minutes (including freezing time)

Cooking Time: 45 minutes

Ingredients for Base Layer

- Erythritol, ½ cup

- Coconut flour (sifted), 1 cup

- Ground ginger, 1 ¼ tsp

- Baking cocoa powder (unsweetened), 1 tbsp

- Baking soda, ½ tsp

- Ground nutmeg, ¼ tsp

- Salt, ½ tsp

- Coconut oil, ½ cup

- 2 Eggs

- Pure vanilla extract, 2 tsp

Ingredients for Cheese Layer

- 1 large egg

- Pure pumpkin puree, ½ cup

- Cream cheese (softened), 8 oz.

- Erythritol, ¼ cup

- Ground nutmeg, a pinch

- Ground ginger, ¼ tsp

- Ground cinnamon, ½ tsp

Directions

1. Set the oven to preheat setting at 350 degrees F. Prepare a 8 x 8 baking pan and grease it.

2. In a large mixing bowl, add all the dry ingredients for the base layer and whisk together to combine well.

3. Add eggs, oil, and vanilla to the dry mixture and continue to mix until it becomes crumbly and stiff.

4. Separate one cup of this mixture for the topping and press the remaining in the baking pan. Use a spatula to firmly press down and tighten the layer. Set aside and prepare the cheesecake layer.

5. Add all the cheesecake ingredients in a mixing bowl and whisk until well combined. Spread the mixture over the base layer and use a spatula to smooth it out on the top.

6. Top the cheesecake with the remaining crumbly mixture you reserved. Set to bake.

7. Bake for 25-30 minutes until the cheesecake begins to turn slightly brown from the edges. Do not overbake.

8. When done, remove from the oven and place it on a wire rack to let cool. When it is cool enough to handle, cut it in 16 equal bars and remove from the pan. Set to refrigerate for 2 hours to chill.

9. The leftover cheesecake can be stored in the refrigerator for a week.

<u>No-Bake Cashew Bars</u>

Nutrition Information (Per Serving)

- Calories 189.3

- Fats 17.6g

- Fiber 2.1g

- Net carbs 4g

- Protein 4.4g

Serves: 8

Preparation Time: 2 hours 20 minutes (including freezing time)

Cooking Time: - -

Ingredients

- Almond flour, 1 cup

- Natural maple syrup (sugar free), ¼ cup

- Butter (melted), ¼ cup

- Cinnamon 1 tsp

- Cashews, ½ cup

- Salt, a pinch

- Shredded coconut, ¼ cup

Directions

1. Add almond flour and melted butter in a large mixing bowl and combine.

2. Add maple syrup, salt, cinnamon, and shredded coconut to the mixture and mix well.

3. Chop cashews roughly and add into the dough. Fold all the ingredients together.

4. Prepare a baking sheet and line it with parchment paper. Spread the dough and smooth it out with a spatula.

5. Set to refrigerate for 2 hours until chilled.

6. Slice into bars and serve chilled for delicious cashew bars!

Peanut Butter Tart

Nutrition Information (Per Serving)

- Calories 304.8

- Fats 26.8g

- Fiber 6.6g

- Net carbs 3.9g

- Protein 9.8g

Serves: 4

Preparation Time: 2 hours 10 minutes (including refrigerating time)

Cooking Time: 10 minutes

Ingredients for crust

- Flaxseeds (flaxseed meal), ¼ cup

- Erythritol, 1 tbsp

- Almond oil, 2 tbsp

- 1 large egg white

Ingredients for Top Layer

- Cocoa powder, 4 tbsp

- 1 medium avocado

- Cinnamon, ½ tsp

- Vanilla extract, ½ tsp

- Heavy cream, 2 tbsp

Ingredients for Middle Layer

- Butter, 2 tbsp

- Peanut butter, 4 tbsp

Directions

1. Set the oven to preheat setting at 350 degrees F.

2. To prepare crust, use flaxseed meal or grind ¼ cup of flaxseeds.

3. Add remaining crust ingredients to the flaxseed meal and combine thoroughly.

4. When the crust mixture is prepared, press it down on tart pans and on the sides. Set to bake for 8-10 minutes until totally set.

5. Remove from oven and set aside to let cool.

6. Melt butter and peanut butter in a pan or microwave until soft. Mix well and pour this layer on top of the crust and set to refrigerate for 30 minutes until the soft layer is set.

7. Now combine the chocolate and avocado and set this layer on top of the butter layer. Smooth it out with a spatula or knife.

8. Set to refrigerate again for 30 minutes.

9. Cut slices and serve chilled!

Chocolate Roll Cake

Nutrition Information (Per Serving)

- Calories 274.2

- Fats 25.1g

- Fiber 3.9g

- Net carbs 2.8g

- Protein 5.8g

Serves: 12

Preparation Time: 30 minutes

Cooking Time: 15 minutes

Ingredients for Chocolate Roll

- Butter (melted), 4 tbsp

- Almond flour, 1 cup

- 3 eggs

- Cocoa powder, ¼ cup

- Psyllium husk powder, ¼ cup

- Coconut milk, ¼ cup

- Erythritol, ¼ cup

- Sour cream, ¼ cup

- Vanilla, 1 tsp

- Baking powder, 1 tsp

Ingredients for Cream Cheese Filling

– Cream cheese, 8 oz.

– Sour cream, ¼ cup

– Butter, 8 tbsp

– Stevia, ¼ tsp

– Vanilla, 1 tsp

Directions

1. In a large mixing bowl, add all the dry ingredients and mix well.

2. Add wet ingredients to the dry mixture one by one and keep folding in.

3. Mix until it forms a dough-like texture. Spread it out on a silpat on cookie sheet and smooth on top.

4. Set to bake at 350 degrees F for 12-15 minutes. When the cake is done, remove and let chill for a while.

5. Meanwhile, prepare the cream cheese filling. Combine all the ingredients of cream cheese together in a mixing bowl.

6. Spread filling on the thin cake layer evenly and roll it up tightly.

7. Cut slices and set to refrigerate.

8. Serve chilled and enjoy!

Pecan Muffins

Nutrition Information (Per Serving)

- Calories 208

- Fats 20.7g

- Fiber 2.8g

- Net carbs 1.5g

- Protein 4.8g

Serves: 11

Preparation Time: 20 minutes

Cooking Time: 30 minutes

Ingredients

- Pecan halves, ¾ cup

- Almond flour, 1 cup

- Red mill golden flaxseed, ½ cup

- Coconut oil, ½ cup

- Erythritol, ¼ cup

- 2 eggs

- Maple extract, 2 tsp

- Baking soda, ½ tsp

- Vanilla extract, 1 tsp

– Apple cider vinegar, ½ tsp

– Liquid stevia, ¼ tsp

Directions

1. Set oven to preheat setting at 325 degrees F.

2. Add pecan halves into a food processor and pulse to chop. Remove from processor and separate 2/3rd portion. Leave 1/3 nuts to use later.

3. In another bowl, add all wet ingredients and combine well.

4. Combine all the remaining dry ingredients with chopped pecans. Add wet mixture to the dry mixture and fold it in.

5. Prepare a muffin tray and add liners to it. Distribute the batter into the tins and top with the remaining chopped pecans.

6. Set to bake for 25-30 minutes until done.

7. Remove from oven and let cool before serving.

8. Enjoy fresh flavors!

These are some delicious, hand-picked recipes that you can enjoy. Don't forget to mark your favorite ones to try whenever you like!

Chapter 4: What An Ideal Ketogenic Meal Plan Should Look Like

The whole idea to follow is to get full on fats from morning until the dinner. The myriad of benefits have already been discussed above. While the entire plan is easy to understand, it could be a little difficult to follow without a schedule. Thus, it is important that you design one by further understanding what should be expected from you for breakfast, lunch, and dinner when you are following the diet.

One thing you need to make sure is to adjust your eating time. Setting the same time to eat every day will keep you active and will fix your eating schedule. The ideal time to have your breakfast is 7am and serve dinner by 7pm. These two meals should be clearly 12 hours apart. This will keep your body in the ideal fasted state.

This is a state where the body is able to break down extra-fat that is stored in the body for energy. Set your lunch time in between these 12-hour break– ideally 1 pm –to set your body's clock accordingly.

This is where things will start falling into place and will become fun. The best part? You now have these amazing recipes to start with.

Breakfast

You can go full on with fats for breakfast time – try out some of the breakfast recipes mentioned above. Instead of doubling the amount of tea or coffee, focus on doubling the amount of butter, coconut oil, and heavy cream.

It should also have an impact on the amount of calories but the best part is that it should be enough to keep you satiated all the way to dinner. However, you do not necessarily have to skip lunch. You can pick a relatively lighter option for lunch time.

Also, don't forget to continue drinking water throughout the day to keep yourself hydrated.

Lunch

You can pick any option from the lunch menu – preferably the lighter ones –to fill yourself up if you are not hungry. Whatever you eat will help you feel energized and full all the way until the dinner time.

Serve yourself a delicious beverage from the options above and keep drinking water to make sure you are staying hydrated.

Dinner

You can go a little overboard with dinner, especially if you have skipped the meal. The dinner will stay the same. Don't hesitate in enjoy your meats, fats, and vegetables.

Also, enjoy one dessert per week.

Food, treats, sweets, and losing weight – that's a lucky weight loss program, no?

The ketogenic diet is undoubtedly a great method for losing weight without really compromising on the food and flavors.

This diet is not only going to help you with weight loss but will also help you with fixing a lot of health problems.

So get started with it today, fight obesity, enjoy food and recipes, and get on the journey of weight loss today!

Conclusion

As mentioned earlier, Ketogenic is not a diet, but a lifestyle. It is a way of changing your eating patterns to minimize the intake of carb to achieve maximum health benefits – including weight loss.

The book included details and great information about how you can prepare yourself for this change and the steps you needed to consider before making your final decision. So, I hope it was able to help you get started with the Ketogenic lifestyle...

The next step is to prepare your mind, read the book again and again, follow a plan that helps you follow one step at a time and prepare some delicious recipes that makes you stick to this diet plan.

If you have tried a thousand ways to lose weight without success, this is your best time to start. If you do this, by the same time next week, you will be several pounds lighter, thanks to this amazing diet—and week after week you will be a healthier and lighter version of who you are now.

Try out the amazing recipes and go through the shopping list to find out what you will need in your pantry to keep up with your healthy lifestyle. Mark your favorite recipes and get started now!

Again, THANK YOU for buying my book; I hope you enjoyed reading it as much as I enjoyed writing it!

And one last thing...

...I Need Your Help!

I would love to hear what you thought of my book. I would honestly, wholeheartedly, appreciate it if you left an honest review for me on Amazon.

Thank you and I wish you all the best as you embark on your health journey... May you have great health and motivation as you seek to find health and joy with the help of the Ketogenic diet!

Preview Of "Mediterranean Diet: A Simple Cookbook & Guide For Busy People To Rapid Weight Loss & Healthy Eating Mastery"

Mastering the Mediterranean Diet
Where It All Began

The varied cuisines of the Mediterranean have developed over the millennia, with notable regional changes happening with the introduction of New World foods starting in the 16th century. The concept of a Mediterranean cuisine, however, is very recent. Although it was first publicized in 1945 by the American doctor Ancel Keys stationed in Salerno, Italy, the Mediterranean diet failed to gain widespread recognition until the 1990s. Our collective obsession with the Mediterranean diet and lifestyle began in the late 1950s when scientists noticed that Spain, Italy, Southern France, Greece and Turkey experienced far fewer deaths from heart disease than most other countries in the world. They eventually determined that low intakes of saturated fat were one of the diet's features that protected the hearts of people in the region. Objective data showing that the Mediterranean diet is healthy, first originated from the Seven Countries Study. The Mediterranean diet is based on what from the point of view of mainstream nutrition is considered a paradox: that although the people living in Mediterranean countries tend to consume relatively high amounts of fat, they have far lower rates of cardiovascular disease than in countries like the United States, where similar levels of fat consumption arefound.

A number of diets have received attention, but the strongest evidence for a beneficial health effect and decreased mortality after switching to a largely plant based diet comes from studies of Mediterranean diet, e.g. from the NIH-AARP Diet and Health Study. The Mediterranean diet is often cited as beneficial for being low in saturated fat and high in monounsaturated fat and dietary fiber. One of the main explanations is thought to be the health effects of olive oil included in the Mediterranean diet. The Mediterranean diet is high in salt content.Foods such as olives, salt-cured cheeses, anchovies, capers, salted fish roe, and salads dressed with extra virgin olive oil all contain high levels of salt. The inclusion of red wine is considered a factor contributing to health as it contains flavonoids with powerful antioxidant properties.

Benefits Of The Diet

Here's what science has to say about the positive effects of the eating habits of Mediterranean natives:

Keeps elders agile:

A 2012 study conducted on elderly residents of Tuscany, Italy, found that keeping to a Mediterranean-style diet decreased a senior's odds of developing hallmark signs of frailty (slow walking speed, muscle weakness, generalized exhaustion) by about 70 percent, when compared to those who subscribed to a different nutritional program. Avoiding signs of frailty can help prevent falls, fractures and broken bones in the elderly.

Fights chronic ailments:

Study after study shows how Mediterranean diet foods can help reduce a person's risk for developing chronic illnesses, including heart disease, diabetes, cancer, arthritis, dental disease, macular degeneration and Alzheimer's. They may also play a role in helping people with asthma and chronic obstructive pulmonary disease (COPD) manage their condition.

Visit www.Amazon.com to check out the rest of "Mediterranean Diet: A Simple Cookbook & Guide For Busy People To Rapid Weight Loss & Healthy Eating Mastery", as well as other books by Lilly Fitt.

Other Books By Lilly Fitt

Below you'll find some of my other popular books that are popular on Amazon and Kindle as well.

Mediterranean Diet: The Busy People Guide To Weight Loss

Alternatively, you can visit my author page on Amazon to see other work done by me. More and more are coming out all the time, so connect with me to receive updates of my new work!

Visit my Amazon Author Page here:

https://www.amazon.com/Lilly-Fitt/e/B01GPYAT6Y

www.ingramcontent.com/pod-product-compliance
Lightning Source LLC
Chambersburg PA
CBHW070144290526
45789CB00002B/622